# Copyright

Table of contents

## Introduction

A. Importance of exercise for seniors:

As we journey through life, our bodies experience natural changes, mainly as we enter our golden years. It becomes increasingly necessary to put our health and well-being first. For seniors over the age of 60, exercise isn't just about remaining in shape; it's about maintaining sovereignty, boosting overall quality of life, and promoting liveliness.

B. **Benefits of exercising at home:**

In the modern world, the convenience of exercising at home has never been more enticing or accessible. While the prospect of going to the gym may seem frightening, building a comfortable workout area within your own home offers an attractive option. Exercising at home eliminates many of the barriers that may dissuade seniors from being active, such as transportation issues, financial worries, or time limits. It allows you to workout on your own terms, at your own pace, and in a familiar, comfortable setting.

## C. **Target audience and goals of the book:**

This book is designed with a specific audience in mind: **seniors aged 60 and above** who are keen to embrace a healthier, more active lifestyle. Our primary goal is to empower you with the knowledge and resources to go on a journey of physical fitness that is safe, pleasurable, and sustainable. We'll lead you through a complete program of easy home workouts that cater to your individual requirements and limits, offering the support and motivation you need to succeed.

Throughout the next chapters, we will cover a wide range of issues, from assessing your current fitness level and setting realistic objectives to creating a safe exercise area at home. You'll discover the value of warming up and including easy stretching exercises, explore low-impact cardiovascular exercises intended to boost heart health, and learn essential tools for tracking your progress.

We'll delve into the world of strength and balance workouts, providing you with crucial instruction on preserving muscle health and preventing falls. Flexibility and mobility exercises can help keep you limber and active, and we'll give you sample exercise routines that you may customize to your unique needs.

Your total well-being isn't just dependent on exercise, so we'll look into the crucial parts of diet and hydration that complement your fitness journey. And when obstacles emerge, as they surely will, this book will provide you with ways to conquer them, from managing aches and pains to staying motivated and getting medical help when necessary.

We'll also discuss the social and emotional benefits of exercise, including its positive impact on mental health and the opportunity to develop a supportive network of like-minded individuals. As we complete our trip together, and stay active and healthy well beyond the age of 60.

This book is not simply a handbook; it's an invitation to embrace a more lively, fulfilling, and healthy existence. By the time you reach the last chapter, our objective is that you'll be armed with the information, inspiration, and practical tools needed to embark on a lifelong commitment to fitness and well-being. Additionally, we've included appendices with activity tracking sheets, recipes for senior-friendly meals, and a glossary of terms to guide you on your path. With this thorough guide by your side, you'll be well on your way to accomplishing your fitness goals and enjoying the myriad benefits that come with an active, healthy lifestyle.

# Chapter 1

## Getting Started

A. **Evaluating Your Fitness Level:**

Before commencing any exercise program, it's necessary to examine your present fitness level. This initial step acts as a basis for your fitness journey and helps adapt your routines to your unique goals and capabilities. Here's how to assess your fitness level:

Consult your healthcare provider: Start by scheduling a check-up with your healthcare practitioner, especially if you have underlying health disorders or concerns. They can provide valuable insights into your physical state and any workout limits.

Self-Assessment: Evaluate your general health, mobility, and physical skills. Consider factors such as balance, flexibility, strength, and endurance. Take note of any pain or discomfort you may have during your daily activities.

Keep a Healthy Journal: Maintain a record of your medical history, including any prescriptions, surgeries, or injuries. This information will be valuable for both you and your healthcare professional in creating your fitness regimen.

## B. **Setting realistic objectives:**

Setting feasible exercise objectives is vital for motivation and progress tracking. Here's how to develop realistic goals:

Define Your Objectives: Determine what you want to achieve with your fitness routine. It could be enhancing your cardiovascular health, boosting flexibility, growing muscle, or simply remaining active.

Be specific and measurable. Make your goals specific and measurable. For example, strive to walk for 30 minutes five days a week, or enhance your flexibility by being able to touch your toes easily.

progressive advancement: Set goals that allow for progressive advancement. Start with achievable short-term goals, then, as you build confidence and strength, move on to more ambitious ambitions.

Consider timeframes: Decide on a reasonable timetable for reaching your goals. Remember that fitness is a lifelong endeavor, and there's no rush to attain your objectives.

C. **Creating a Safe Exercise Space at Home**: Exercising at home provides convenience and comfort, but safety is vital.

Ensure your exercise space is safe. Clear the area: Remove any barriers or hazards from your workout location.

Make sure there's an adequate area for mobility, especially if you're practicing workouts that entail stretching or balance.

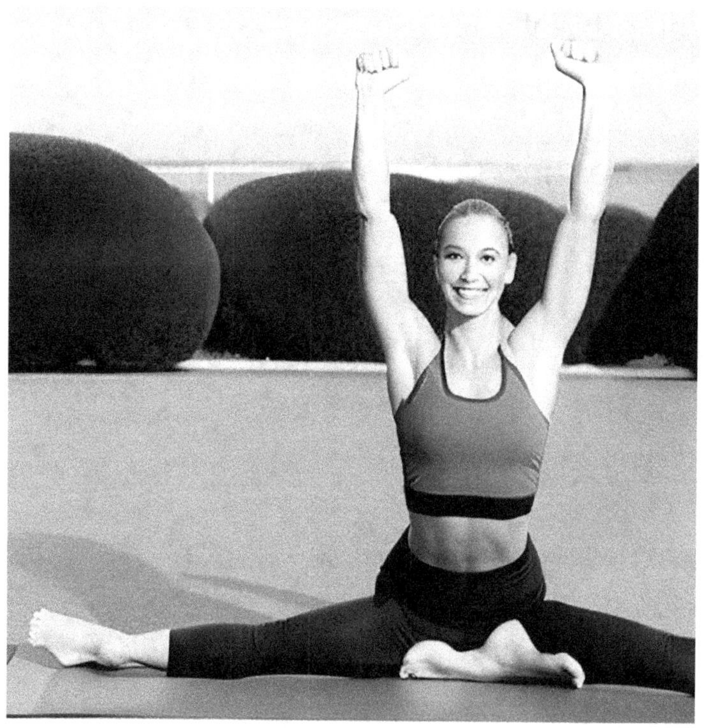

Proper Flooring: Use a non-slip floor or workout mat to prevent slips and falls. This is particularly helpful for activities like yoga or strength training.

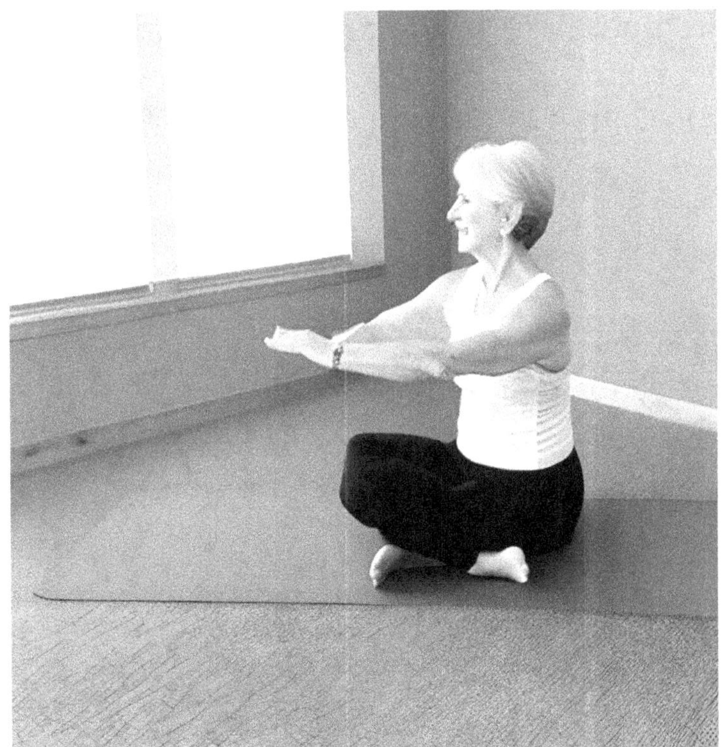

Good Lighting: Ensure your exercise environment is well lit to avoid accidents and maintain visibility during workouts.

Ventilation: Adequate airflow and temperature management are needed to prevent overheating during activity.

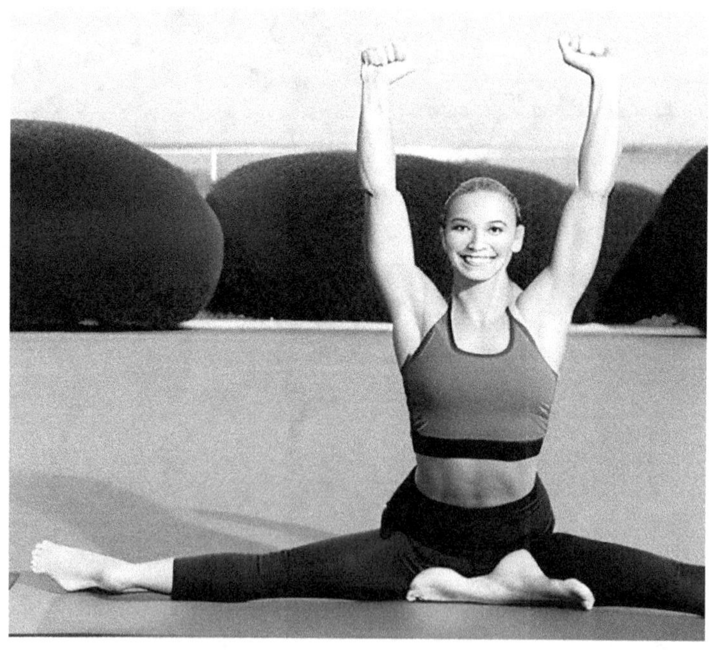

Emergency Preparedness: Keep a phone accessible in case of an emergency, and advise a family member or friend of your exercise program.

D. **Necessary Equipment and Attire:**

You don't need a large array of equipment to exercise at home, but some fundamentals can enhance your workouts:

Comfortable Clothing: Wear breathable, moisture-wicking gear that allows for easy movement. Invest in supportive, comfortable footwear built for your specific activity.

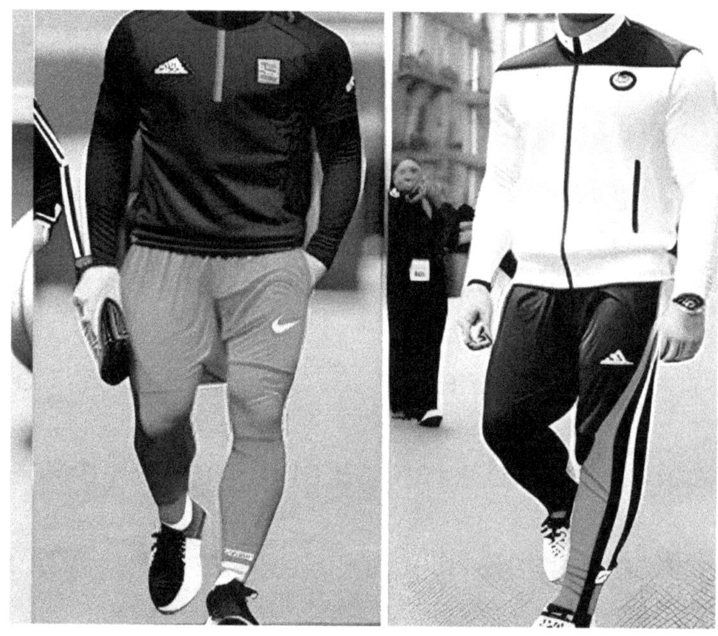

Exercise Mat: A top-quality exercise mat provides padding and support, especially for floor exercises and stretching regimens.

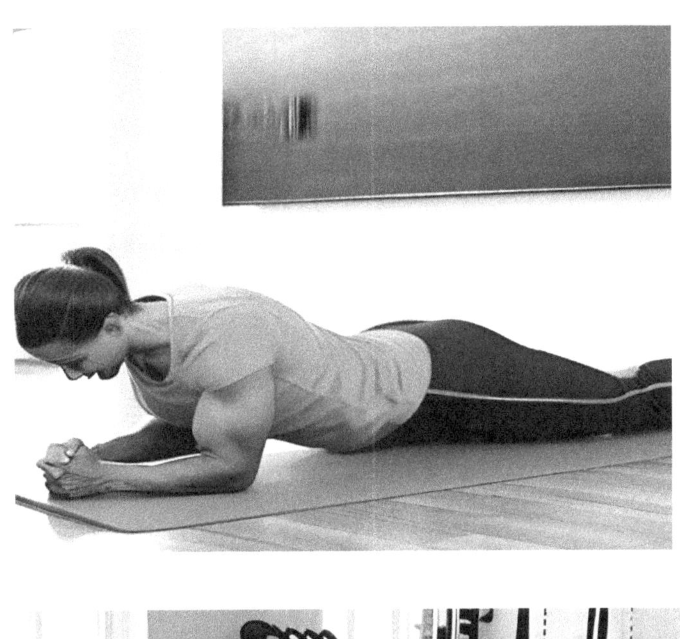

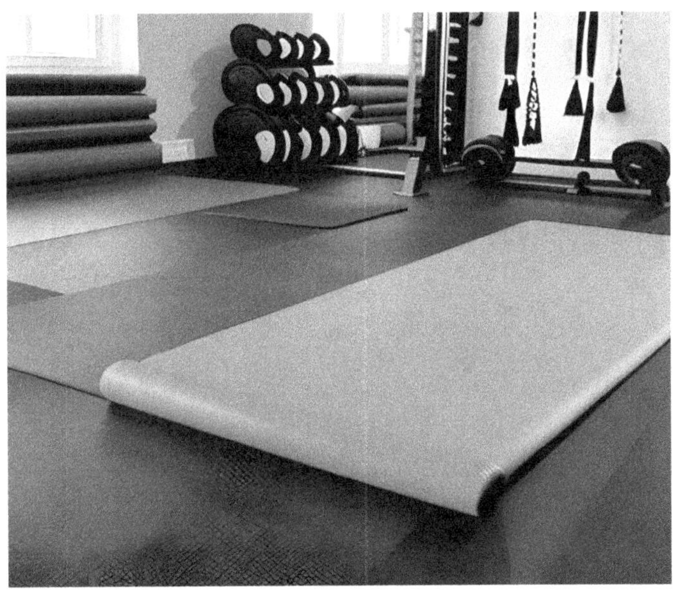

Resistance Bands: These versatile gadgets are good for strength training and are available in varied levels of resistance.

Dumbbells or weights:

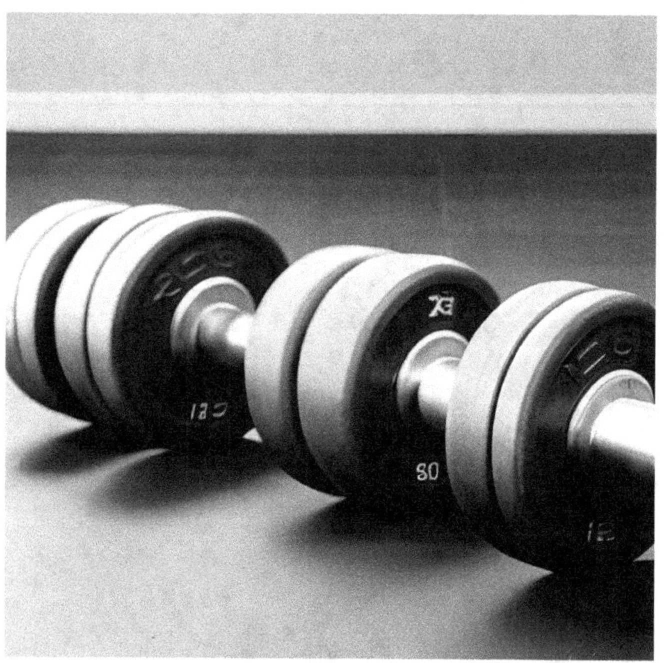

Depending on your fitness goals, having a set of dumbbells or weighted objects might add resistance to your routines.

Timer or stopwatch:

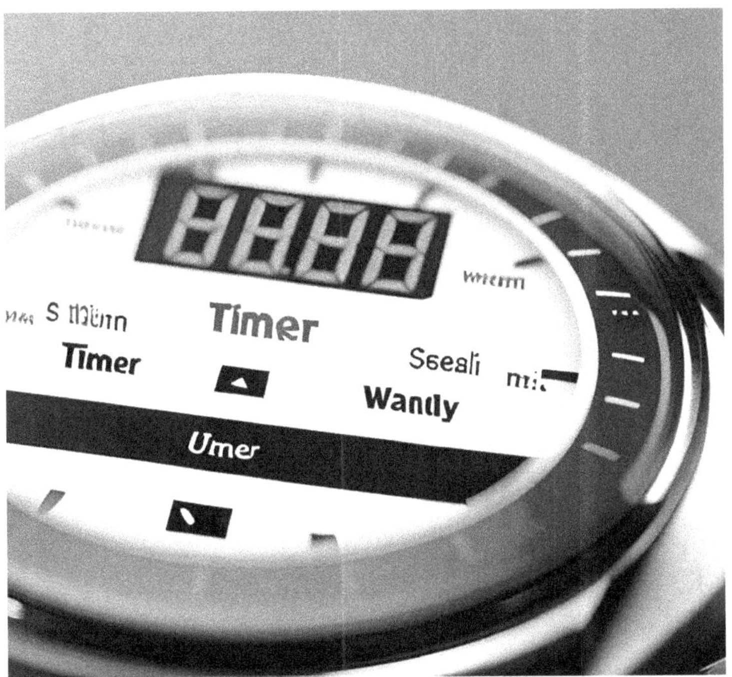

useful for tracking training durations and rest periods.

By measuring your fitness level, setting realistic objectives, creating a safe training environment, and having the required equipment and apparel, you'll be well-prepared to go on your journey to greater health in the comfort of your home. These essential actions will lay the path for successful and pleasurable exercises in the chapters to come.

# Chapter 2:

# Warm-Up and Stretching

## A. **The Importance of Warming Up:**

Warming up is an essential initial step in any workout plan, especially for seniors over 60. Here's why it's so important:

**Injury Prevention**: Warming up gradually boosts your heart rate and blood supply to your muscles. This prepares your body for more intense action and minimizes the likelihood of strains, sprains, and other injuries.

Improved Muscle Function: A proper warm-up helps your muscles become more supple, making them more sensitive to stretching and training. This can increase your overall performance.

**Enhanced Range of Motion**: Warming up gently lubricates your joints, allowing for a larger range of motion during activities. This is particularly beneficial for preserving flexibility as you age.

**Mental Preparation**: It provides a mental transition from ordinary tasks to exercise, helping you focus and get in the correct mood for your workout.

B. **Gentle Stretching Exercises**:

Stretching is an integral component of your warm-up regimen. Gentle stretching activities help promote flexibility, alleviate muscle tension, and prepare your body for physical activity. Here are some recommended gentle stretching exercises:

**Arm and chest stretching**: Extend one arm across your chest and gently grasp it with the other hand. Repeat on both sides.

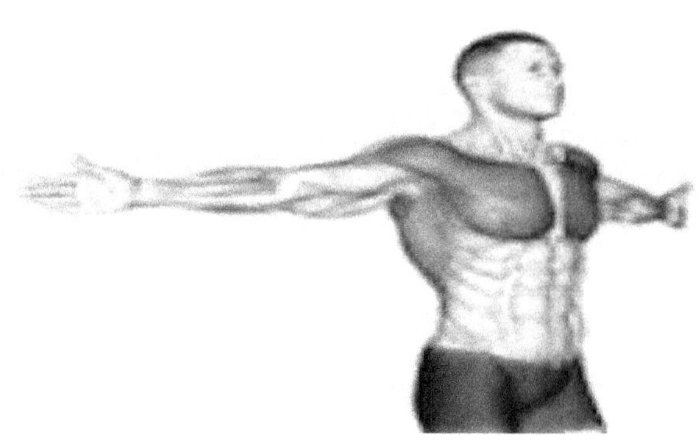

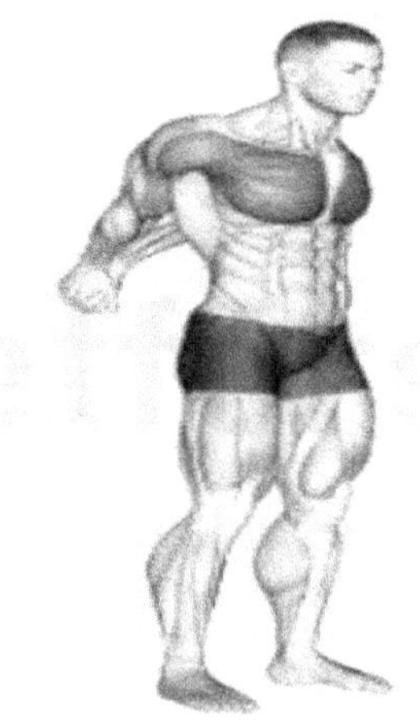

Side Bends:

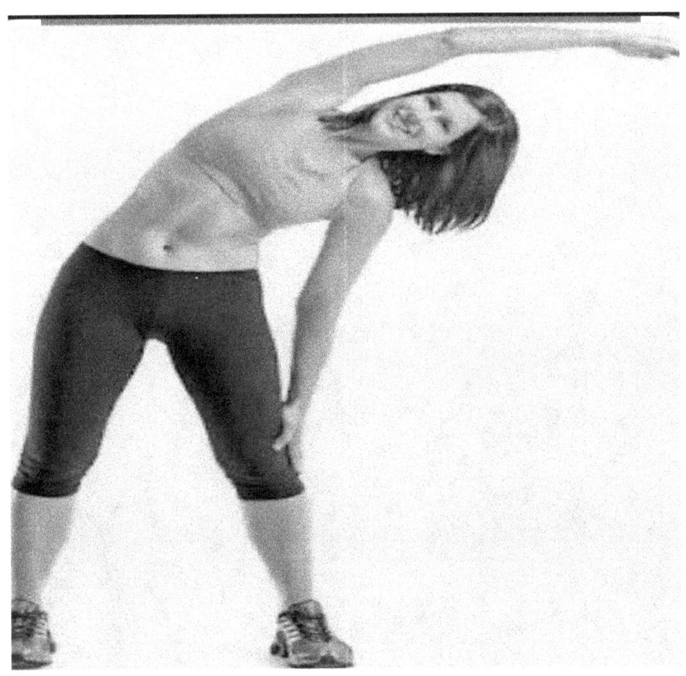

Stand or sit erect, then slowly bend your upper body to the side, stretching your oblique muscles. Alternate sides.

Reach for your toes, keeping your back straight, to stretch your hamstrings and lower back.

Ankle Circles:

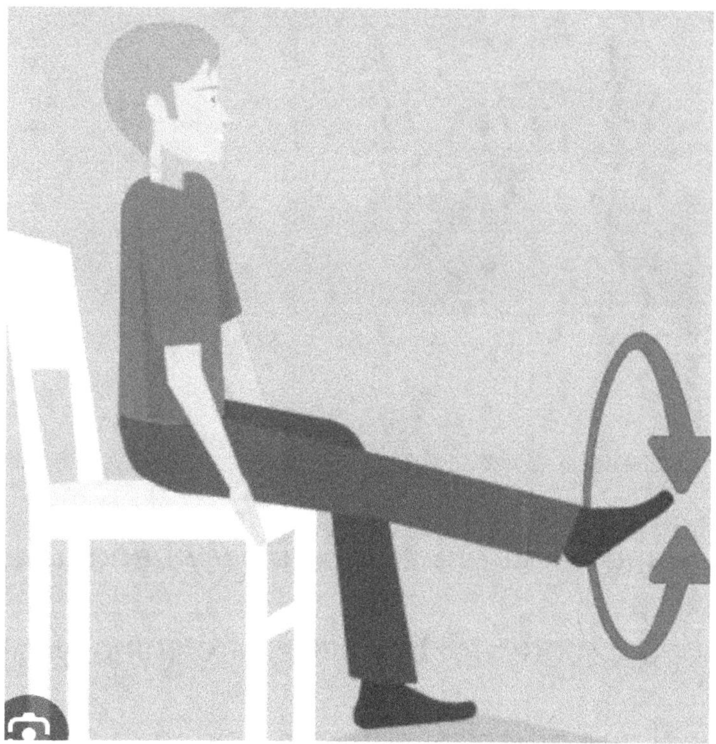

While seated, elevate one foot off the ground and rotate your ankle clockwise and counterclockwise to enhance ankle mobility.

Hip Flexor Stretch:

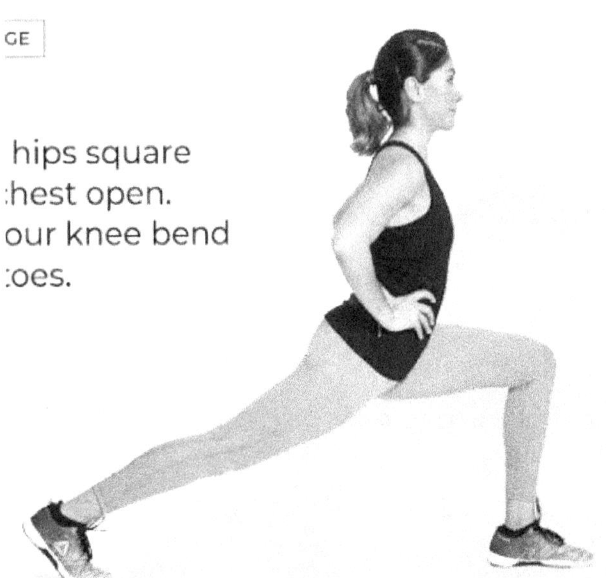

Stand and take a step back with one foot, bending your front knee. Gently lift your hips forward to stretch your hip flexors. Repeat on both sides.

C. **Breathing and Relaxation Techniques:** Incorporating breathing and relaxation techniques into your warm-up will increase your entire exercise experience.

Deep Breathing: Take slow, deep breaths while you complete your stretching activities. Deep breaths can help soothe the nervous system and lessen tension.

Mindful Stretching: Pay attention to the sensations in your body as you stretch. Focus on each muscle group you're targeting and envision them becoming more relaxed and flexible.

Progressive Muscle Relaxation: As you stretch, intentionally release tension from your muscles. Start at your toes and work your way up to your head, relaxing each body part as you go.

Meditation: Incorporate a short meditation session into your warm-up. This can enhance concentration and reduce anxiety, making your exercise regimen more enjoyable.

Remember that your warm-up and stretching regimen should be moderate and progressive, concentrating on ease of movement and comfort. Avoid bouncing or straining your body into positions that create pain. As we age, it's crucial to prioritize safety and listen to our bodies, gradually working up to more rigorous workouts as we progress through the chapters ahead.

# Chapter 3

## Low-Impact Cardiovascular Exercises

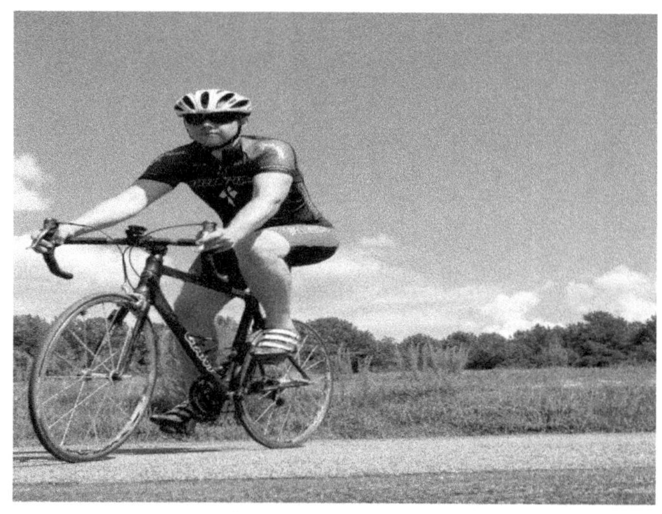

Aerobic Exercises for Heart Health:

Aerobic workouts, generally referred to as "cardio," are a cornerstone of a good fitness routine, especially for seniors over 60. These activities can enhance cardiovascular health, build endurance, and increase overall energy levels. Here are some low-impact aerobic exercises ideal for seniors:

Walking: Brisk walking is a gentle and effective way to get your heart rate up. You can perform this indoors or outdoors, depending on your preference and the weather.

Stationary Cycling:

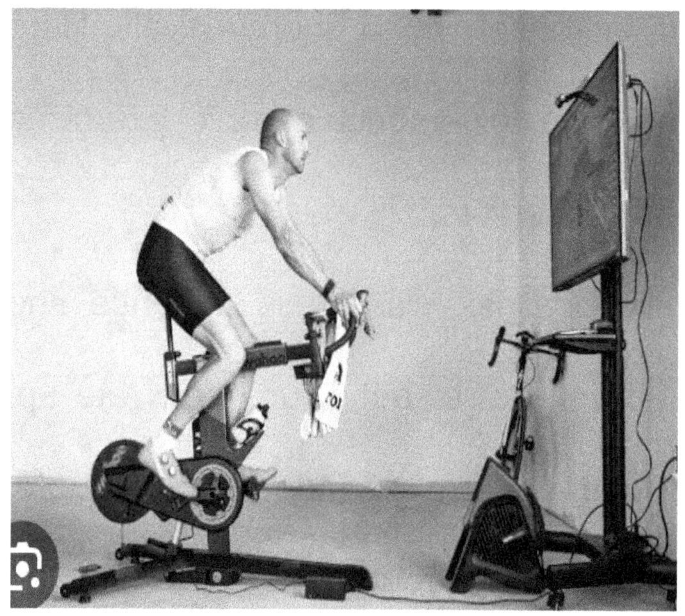

Use a stationary workout bike to get your heart beating without placing excessive stress on your joints.

Swimming or water aerobics: Water provides natural resistance and supports your body, making it a good alternative for low-impact cardio activities.

Dancing: Put on your favorite music and dance around your living room. Dancing not only delivers a wonderful cardio workout but also adds an element of pleasure.

Tai Chi:

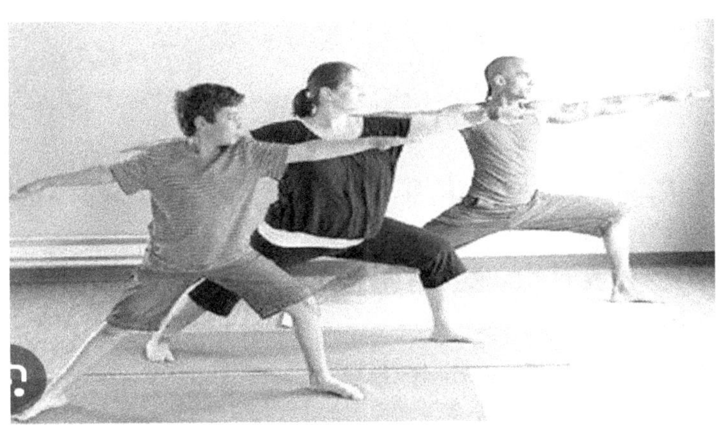

This peaceful martial art blends slow, flowing movements with deep breathing, encouraging balance, flexibility, and cardiovascular health.

Chair Exercises for Lower Body Circulation:

Chair exercises are a terrific alternative for seniors who may have mobility limitations or balance concerns. These exercises can help increase lower body circulation and muscle strength without the need to stand. Here are some chair exercises to consider:

Chair Marches:

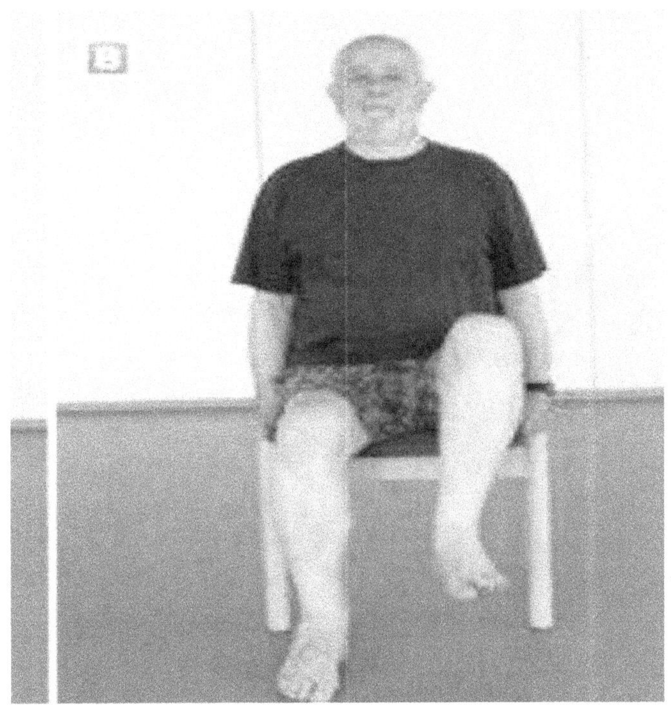

Sit at the edge of a strong chair and lift your knees, one at a time, as if you were marching in place. This movement helps enhance circulation in your legs.

## Chair Leg Lifts:

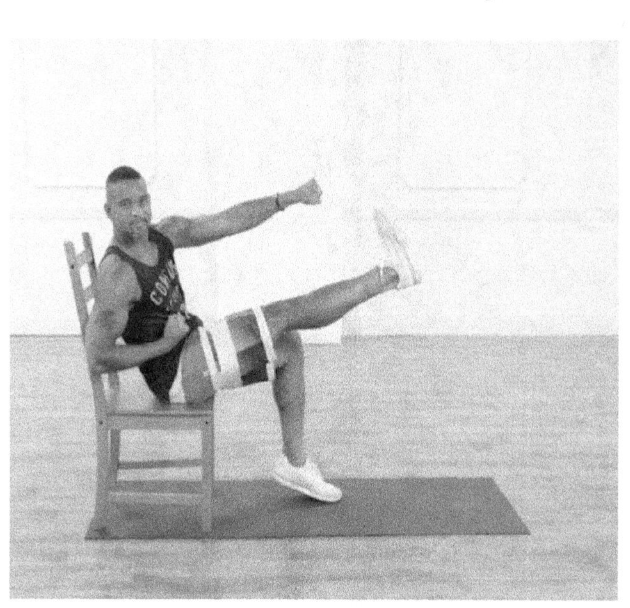

While seated, extend one leg straight in front of you and hold for a few seconds. Lower it down and repeat with the opposite leg. This workout focuses on the quadriceps and builds leg strength.

Chair-Seated Bicycle:

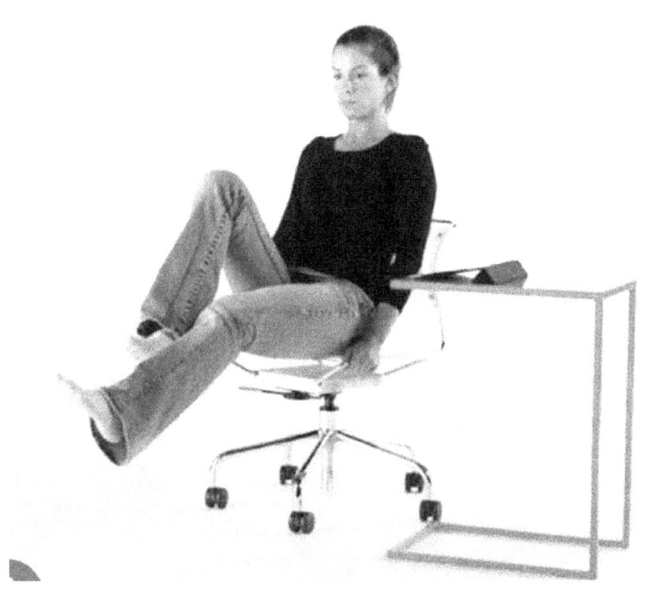

Sit upright in your chair and peddle your legs as if you were riding a bicycle. This activity engages your leg muscles and raises your heart rate.

Chair Tap Dance: Sit with your feet flat on the floor and tap your toes rapidly for 20–30 seconds. This is a great method to boost circulation in your lower legs.

Tracking Progress and Heart Rate Monitoring:

Monitoring your progress is vital to ensuring you're getting the most out of your low-impact cardiovascular activities. Here's how to measure your progress and monitor your heart rate:

Exercise Journal: Keep a journal of your workouts, noting the type of exercise, duration, and any relevant data. This allows you to track improvements over time.

Pulse Check: Periodically check your pulse during your workouts to verify you're in your goal heart rate zone. The optimal heart rate for seniors is normally 50–85% of your maximum heart rate.

Heart Rate Monitor: Consider utilizing a heart rate monitor or fitness tracker. These gadgets provide real-time heart rate data and can help you stay in your desired zone.

Rate of Perceived Exertion (RPE): Use the RPE scale to subjectively rate how hard you feel you're working during exercise. This scale spans from 6 (no exertion) to 20 (highest exertion), with most low-impact cardio routines lying within the 11–14 range for seniors. By including these low-impact cardiovascular workouts into your routine, you can improve your heart health, enhance endurance, and enjoy the many advantages of regular aerobic activity. Monitoring your progress guarantees that you're staying on track and making significant improvements in your fitness quest.

# Chapter 4

## Strength and Balance

Strength Exercises for Muscle Maintenance:


Maintaining muscle strength is vital as we age since it helps promote overall mobility and independence. Here are some strength workouts recommended for elders over 60:

Bodyweight Squats: Stand with your feet shoulder-width apart and lower your body as if you're sitting back into a chair.

Slowly rise back up. This workout strengthens the legs and glutes.

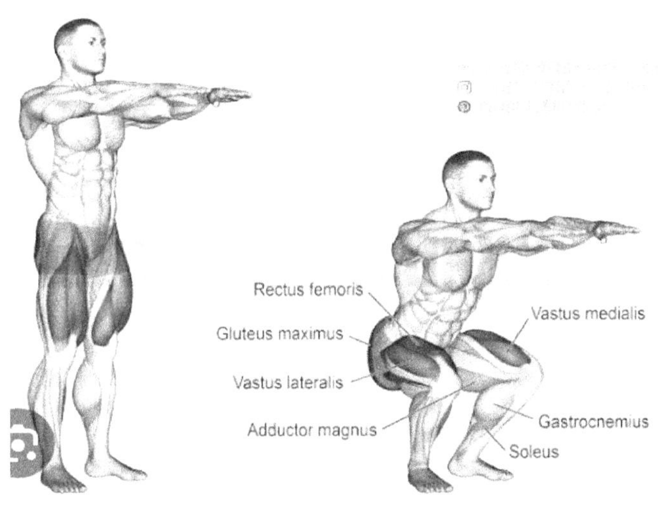


Wall Push-Ups: Stand a few feet away from a wall, place your hands on the wall at shoulder height, and perform push-ups against the wall.

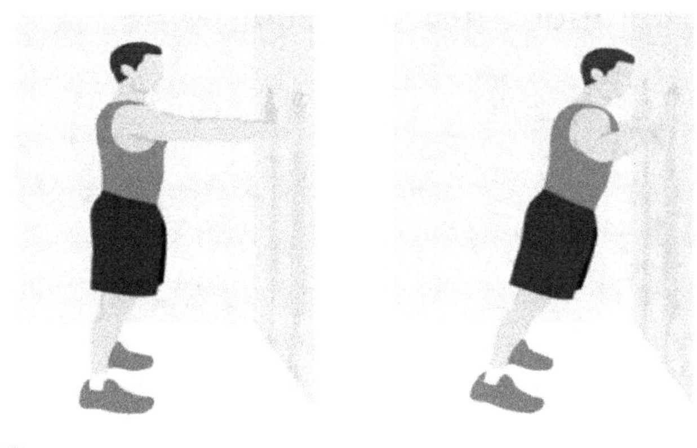

Chair Stand: Sit in a firm chair and stand up without using your hands. Sit back down carefully. This exercise helps strengthen the leg and hip muscles.

Seated Leg Raises:

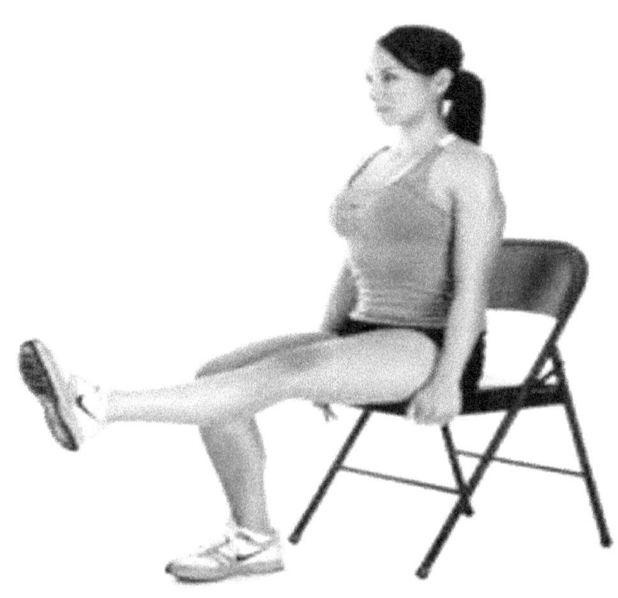

Sit on the edge of a chair and raise one leg straight out in front of you. Hold for a few seconds, and then drop it back down. This workout works the quadriceps.

Resistance band workouts:

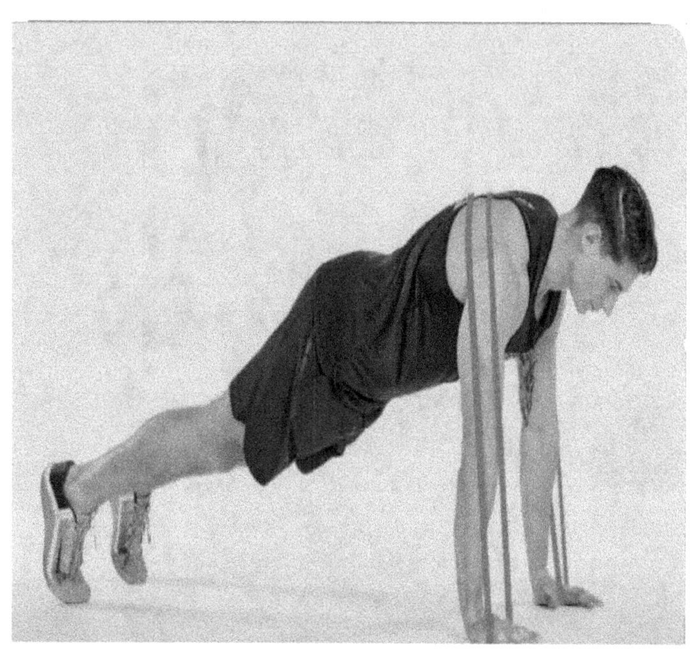

Use resistance bands to do workouts like bicep curls, shoulder presses, and seated rows to target upper body strength.

B. **Balance Exercises to Prevent Falls**:

Maintaining balance is vital for preventing falls, which can have major repercussions for elders. Incorporating balancing exercises into your regimen can help:

Single-Leg Stands:

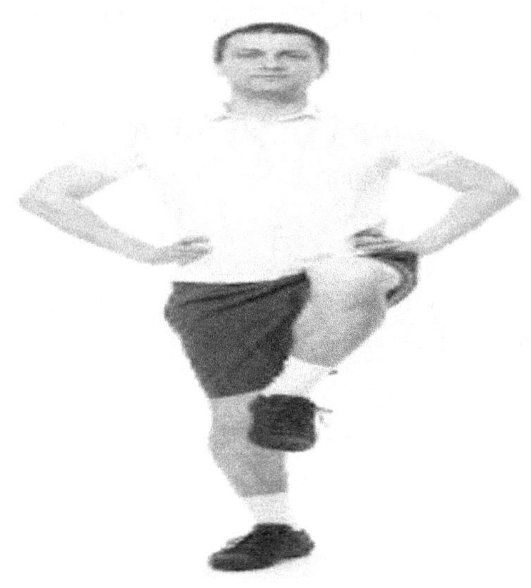

Stand near a sturdy surface (such as a chair or countertop) for support and elevate one leg off the ground. After 10 to 30 seconds, change to the other leg. As you advance, try balancing without support.

Heel-to-toe Walk:

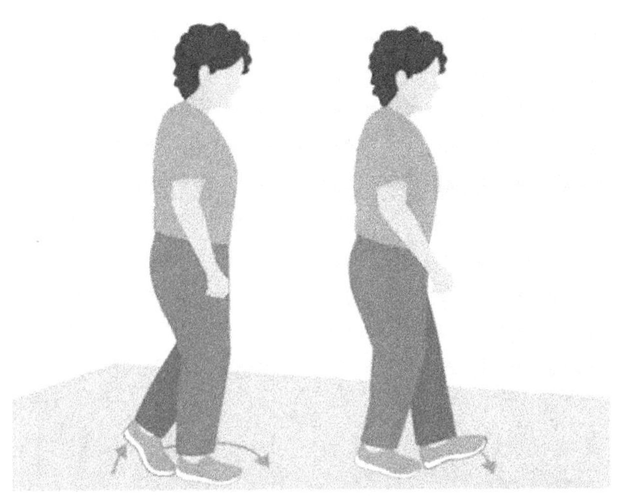

Imagine you're walking on a tightrope. Place one foot directly in front of the other, with your heel touching your toes. Take numerous actions in this manner.

Toe Raises: Stand with your feet hip-width apart and slowly lift your heels off the ground, balancing on your toes.

Lower your heels back down after a few seconds.

Tandem Stance:

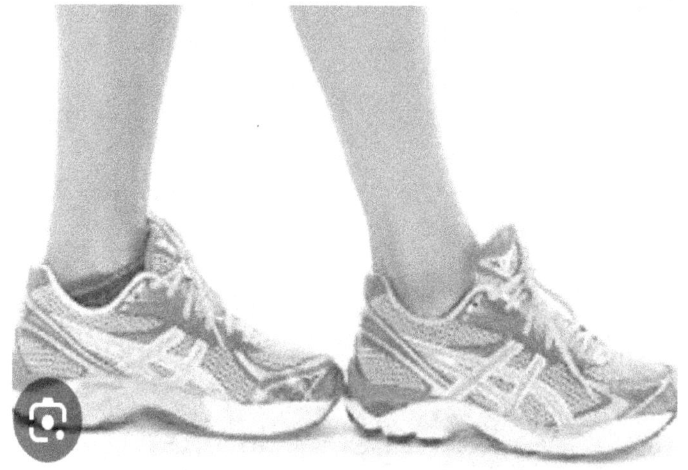

Stand with one foot in front of the other, heel to toe, and hold this stance for as long as you can. Switch the position of your feet after a while.

Balance Games: Consider using balance boards or stability balls for more active balance training. Playing balance games like "standing on one leg while tossing a ball" can help make balance practice more appealing.

C. **Proper Form and Technique**:

Maintaining proper form and technique is critical for both strength and balance exercises.

Start slowly: Begin with exercises that match your current fitness level and progressively improve as you build strength and balance.

Use Correct Posture: Maintain good posture while exercising.

Breathe Properly: Remember to breathe steadily and avoid holding your breath throughout exercises. Proper breathing can help you maintain balance and prevent dizziness.

Stay safe. If you're trying a new workout, consider having a chair or firm surface nearby for support.

Listen to your body. If you encounter pain or discomfort during any workout, stop immediately.

Incorporating strength and balance workouts into your regimen not only helps preserve muscle mass and prevent falls but also contributes to general vitality and well-being. Proper form and technique guarantee that you complete these exercises safely and successfully, receiving the maximum rewards from your efforts.

# Chapter 5

## Flexibility and Mobility:

### Exercises to Improve Flexibility

Flexibility is a fundamental component of general mobility, and it becomes increasingly vital as we age. Incorporating regular flexibility exercises can help you maintain a full range of motion and reduce the chance of injury.

Neck Tilts and Rotations: Gently tilt your head from side to side and rotate it in both directions to increase neck flexibility.

Shoulder Rolls:

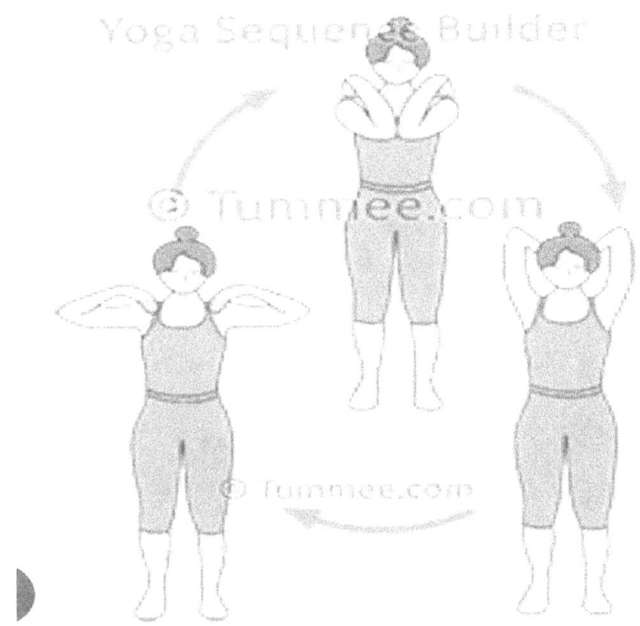

Roll your shoulders forward and backward in a smooth, controlled manner to release tension and promote shoulder flexibility.

Arm and Chest Stretches:

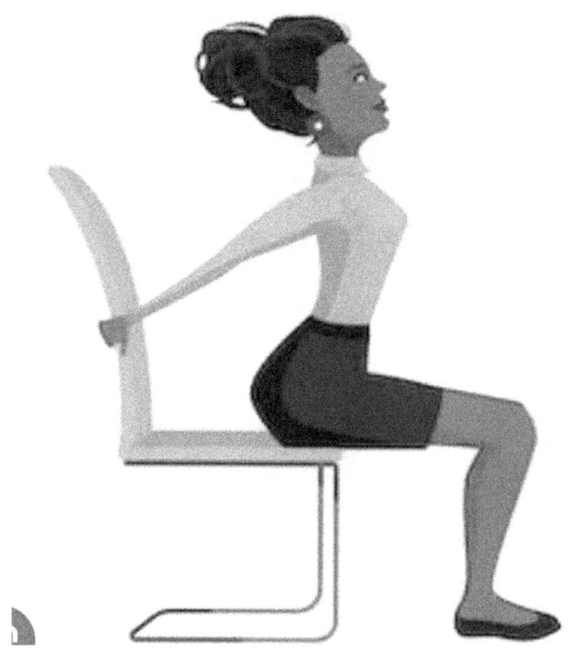

Extend your arms behind your back and clasp your hands together to stretch your chest and shoulders. You can also stretch each arm over your chest.

Back Stretches: Sit or stand up straight, then slowly twist your torso from side to side to stretch your lower back.

Leg Stretches:

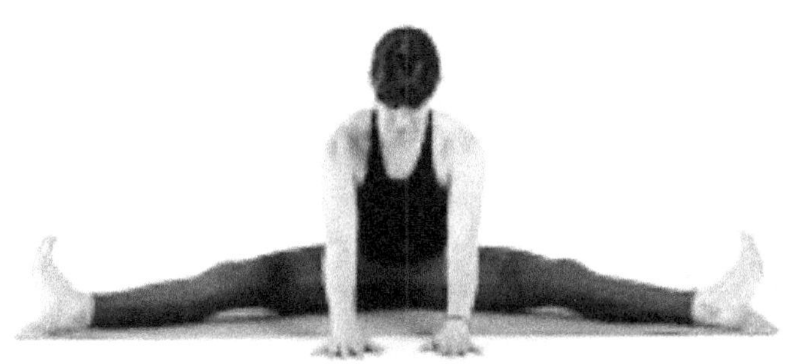

Gentle seated or standing leg stretches help enhance flexibility in your hamstrings, quadriceps, and calf muscles.

Hip Flexor Stretch:

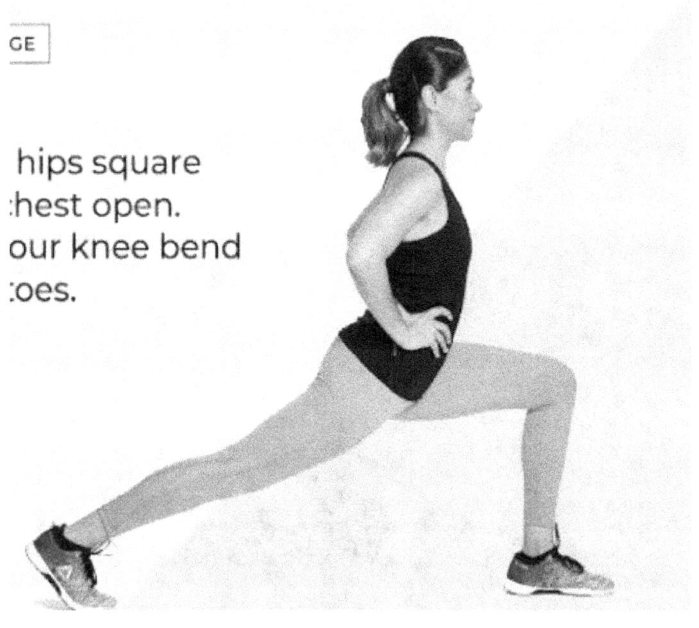



Kneel on one knee and push your hips forward to stretch your hip flexors.

Seated or standing forward Bend: Slowly bend at the hips, reaching towards your toes while keeping your back straight.

B. **Tips for Maintaining Joint Mobility**:

Joint mobility is vital for everyday motions and general quality of life. Here are some strategies to help you preserve joint mobility:

**Stay Active:** Regular physical activity, including walking and modest range-of-motion exercises, can help keep your joints mobile.

Stay hydrated. Proper hydration is vital for joint health.

**Warm-Up**: Always warm up before stretching or indulging in any physical exercise. A warm-up boosts blood flow to the joints and minimizes the chance of damage.

**Avoid Prolonged Immobility**: Try not to sit or stand in the same position for lengthy periods. Take breaks to move and stretch.

Use proper ergonomics: Ensure that your workstation and home surroundings are ergonomically pleasant. This decreases tension on your joints during daily activity.

C. **Stretches for Common Problem Parts**:

Certain parts of the body often require extra attention for stretching due to common concerns related to aging. Here are stretches for these issue areas:

Lower Back Stretch: Lie on your back and raise one knee to your chest while maintaining the other leg straight. Hold for a few seconds, then swap legs.

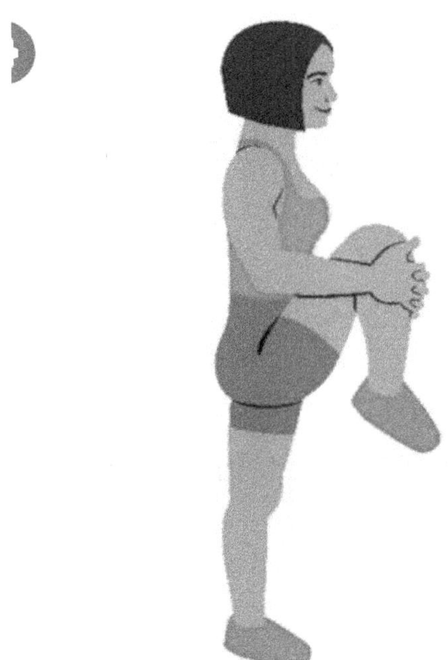

Hip and groin stretch: Sit on the floor with your feet together and gently press your knees toward the ground. This stretch targets the hips and groin.

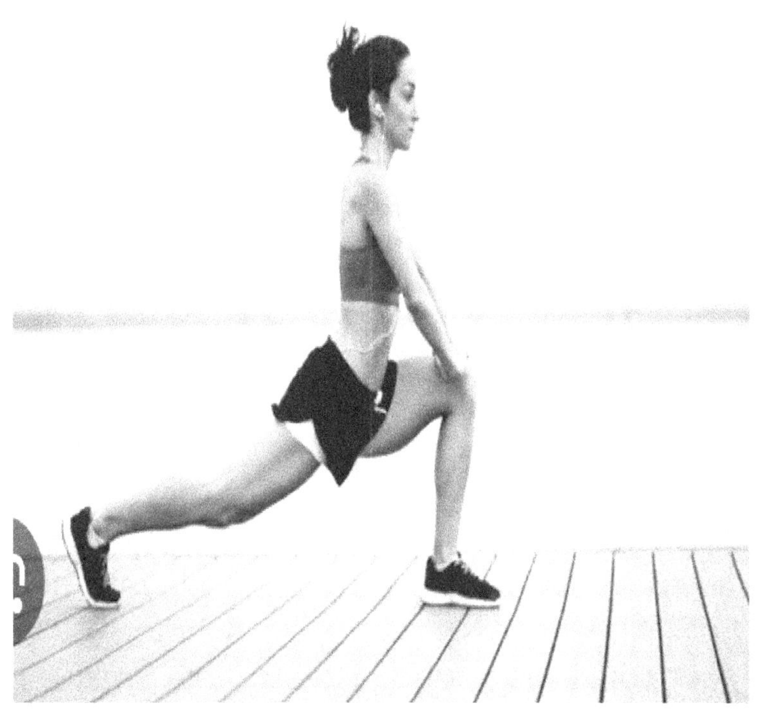

Calf Stretch: Lean against the wall to stretch the calf of the rear leg. Repeat on the other side.

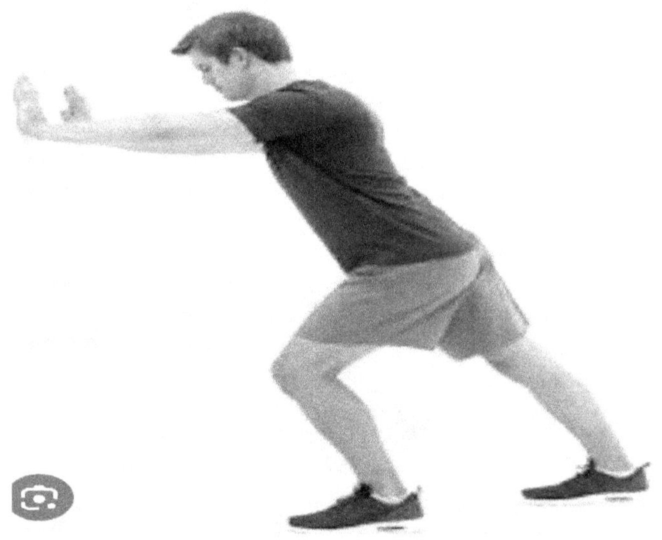

Ankle Circles: Sit down and elevate one leg off the ground. Rotate your ankle in circles to enhance ankle mobility.

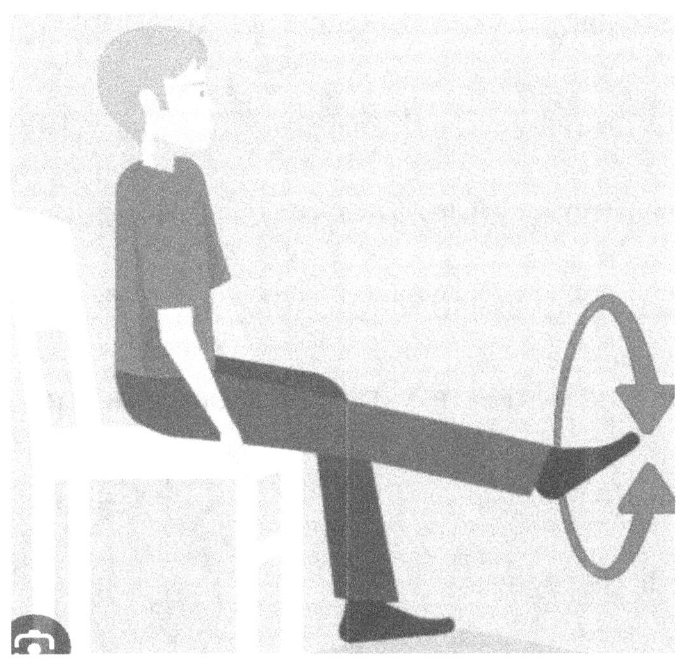

Wrist and Hand Stretch: Extend your arm in front of you, palm facing down. Gently pull your fingers back with your other hand to stretch your wrist and forearm.

Flexibility and mobility are vital for maintaining independence and preventing injury as you age. Regularly executing these stretches and following the guidelines for joint mobility can help you move more freely and comfortably in your daily life.

# Chapter 6

## Exercise Routines:

### A. **Sample Daily and Weekly Exercise Routines:**

Having an organized workout regimen will help you stay consistent and reach your fitness objectives. Here are typical daily and weekly workout routines for adults over 60:

Daily Routine:

**Warm-Up**: Start with 5–10 minutes of mild warm-up exercises, such as neck tilts, shoulder rolls, and ankle circles.

Strength Training: Perform strength exercises 2-3 times a week, targeting different muscle groups on different days. For example, Monday might focus on legs and Thursday on the upper body.

Cardiovascular Exercise: Incorporate low-impact cardio workouts like walking, stationary cycling, or swimming for 20–30 minutes a day, ideally most days of the week.

Flexibility and Mobility: Finish your daily routine with 10–15 minutes of stretching and mobility exercises.

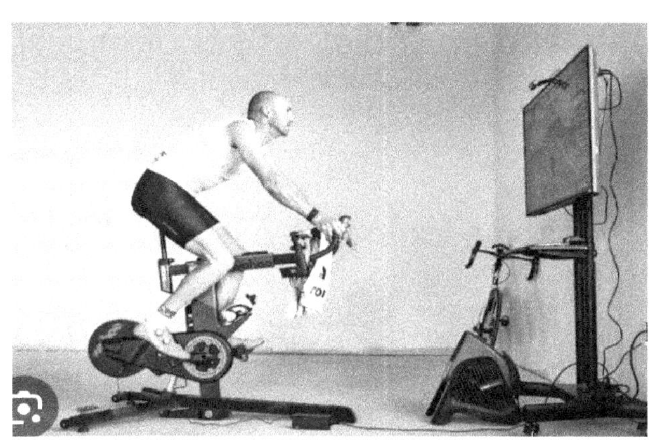

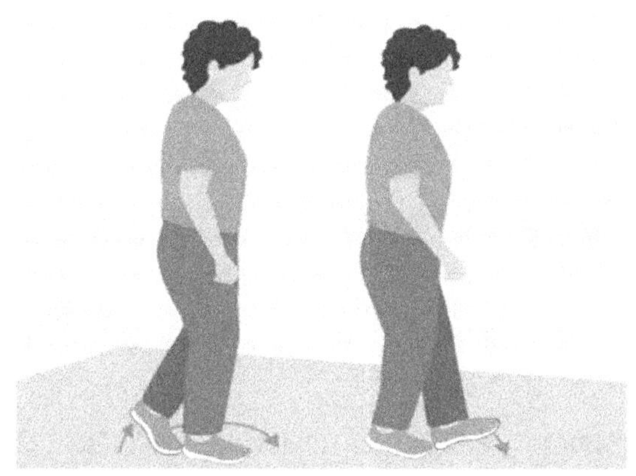

## Weekly Routine:

Strength Training: Include 2-3 days of strength training, each session concentrating on a distinct set of muscle groups.

Cardiovascular Exercise: Aim for at least 150 minutes of moderate-intensity aerobic activity scattered throughout the week. You can break this into smaller sessions if needed.

Flexibility and Mobility: Dedicate 3–4 days to stretching and mobility exercises, addressing various muscle areas each day.

B. Customizing Workouts Based on Individual Needs:

Every individual has unique demands and limits. It's crucial to adapt your workouts to your individual conditions.

Assess your goals: Consider your fitness goals. Do you wish to enhance strength, balance, flexibility, or cardiovascular health? Your goals will determine the types of exercises you prioritize.

Account for Health Conditions: If you have special health issues or conditions, talk with a healthcare physician or physical therapist to establish a workout regimen that accommodates any limitations or restrictions.

Modify Intensity: Adjust the intensity of activities to match your fitness level. Start with lesser resistance or shorter durations and progressively improve as you become more comfortable and capable.

Listen to your body: Pay close attention to how your body responds to each activity. If an activity causes pain or discomfort, adjust or replace it with a more suitable option.

Set realistic expectations. Be realistic about your abilities and growth. It's alright to start small and progressively build up your strength and endurance over time.

Seek Professional Guidance: Consider working with a fitness trainer or physical therapist who specializes in senior fitness. They can provide specialized instruction and ensure your workouts are safe and successful.

C. Incorporating Variety for Continued Motivation:

Maintaining motivation is crucial to continuing with your fitness routine. To keep things new and engaging, include variation in your workouts.

Change workouts regularly: Rotate workouts and vary the types of activities you do to prevent boredom and push different muscle groups.

Try New Activities: Experiment with different forms of exercise, such as yoga,

Pilates, or dancing classes, to keep your routine fresh and exciting.

Set Weekly Challenges: Challenge yourself with weekly goals, such as increasing the duration of your walks or trying a new stretching regimen.

Join a group or class: Participate in group exercise classes or activities with friends or in your community. Social connections can make exercise more enjoyable.

Use technology: Utilize fitness apps or online videos that offer a variety of routines and guided sessions.

Reward Yourself: Celebrate your fitness milestones and triumphs with tiny rewards to maintain a positive attitude towards training.

# Chapter 7

## Nutrition and Hydration:

A. Importance of a Balanced Diet: Nutrition plays a critical role in general health, and for seniors over 60, it's especially crucial. A balanced diet supplies important nutrients, maintains muscle and bone health, and aids in maintaining a healthy weight. Here's why a balanced diet is vital:

## Nutrient-Rich Foods:

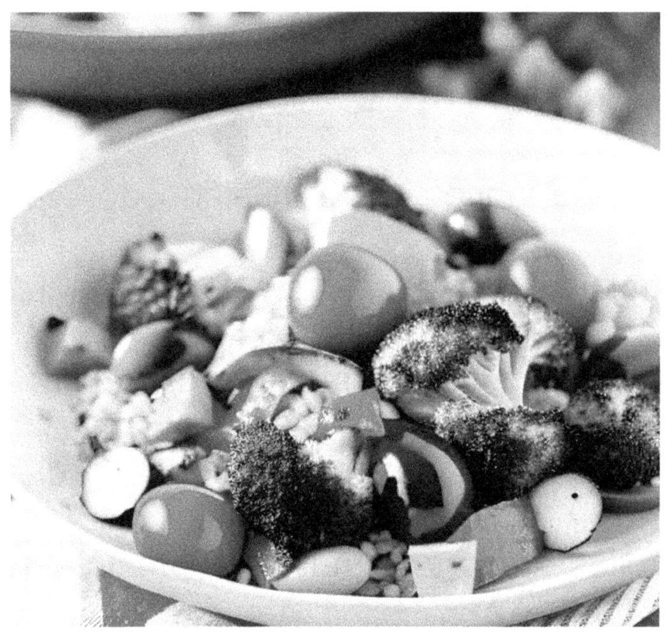

Aim to include a range of nutrient-rich foods in your diet, such as fruits, vegetables, whole grains, lean proteins, and dairy or dairy alternatives. These meals contain critical vitamins and minerals your body needs to function efficiently.

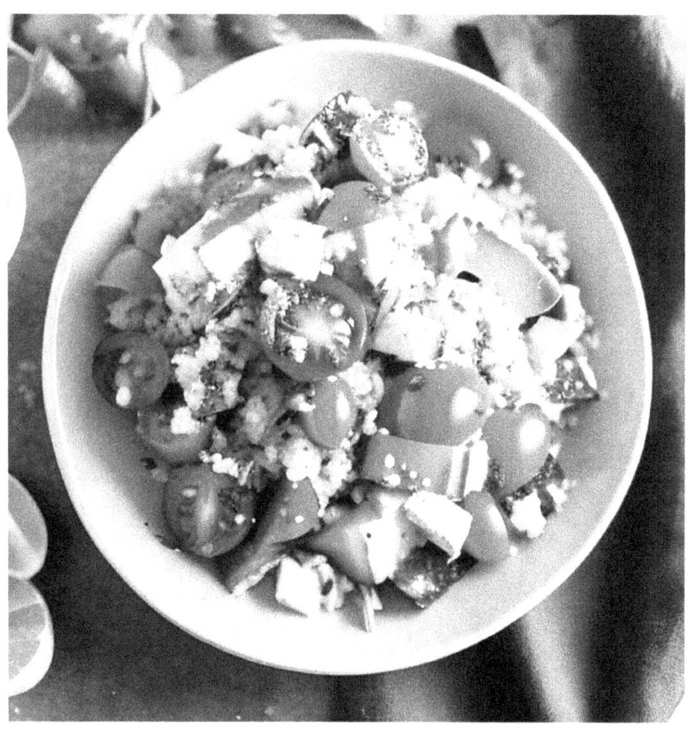

Energy for Exercise: A healthy diet offers the energy necessary for your exercise routines, helping you perform at your best and recuperate effectively.

Muscle Maintenance:

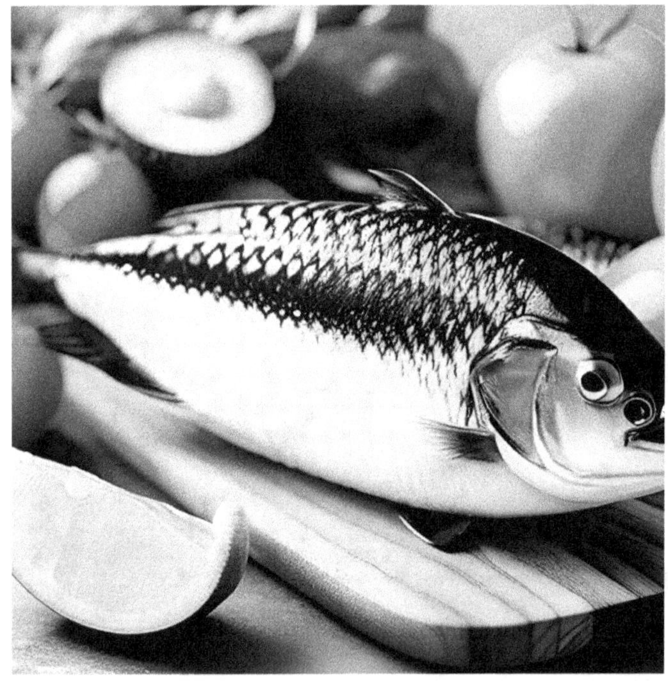

Adequate protein consumption is vital for maintaining muscle mass, which becomes increasingly critical as we age. Incorporate lean protein sources like poultry, fish, legumes, and low-fat dairy into your meals.

Bone Health: Seniors are at greater risk for bone density loss. Calcium-rich foods like dairy products and leafy greens, together with vitamin D from sources like fortified foods and sunlight, are needed for bone health.

Weight Management: A balanced diet helps with weight management by helping you maintain a healthy body weight, which is beneficial for joint health and overall well-being.

B. Hydration Tips for Seniors:

Staying hydrated is crucial, especially as we age. Dehydration can lead to several health complications, including dizziness, urinary tract infections, and constipation.

Drink Water regularly. Don't wait until you feel thirsty, as thirst fades with aging.

Monitor Urine Color: A Pale yellow to light straw tint is a sign of good hydration.

Limit Caffeine and alcohol. These substances can have a diuretic impact, so consume them in moderation. Opt for decaffeinated or herbal beverages wherever feasible.

Stay Hydrated During Exercise: Drink water before, during, and after your workouts, even if you don't feel particularly thirsty.

Include Hydrating Foods: Consume foods with high water content, such as fruits (e.g., watermelon, oranges) and vegetables (e.g., cucumber, lettuce), to contribute to your hydration.

Use a Reusable Water Bottle: Carry a reusable water bottle with you throughout the day as an easy reminder to stay hydrated.

Foods That Support Exercise Goals: Your diet can complement your exercise regimen by delivering the nutrients your body needs for optimal performance and recuperation. Here are some items to include that will assist your workout goals:

Complex Carbohydrates: Foods like whole grains (e.g., brown rice, quinoa, whole wheat pasta) provide long-lasting energy for your workouts.

Lean Proteins: Incorporate lean protein sources including chicken, turkey, fish, tofu, and lentils to help muscle repair and growth.

Healthy Fats: Include sources of healthy fats like avocados, nuts, seeds, and olive oil for prolonged energy and joint health.

Fruits and Vegetables:

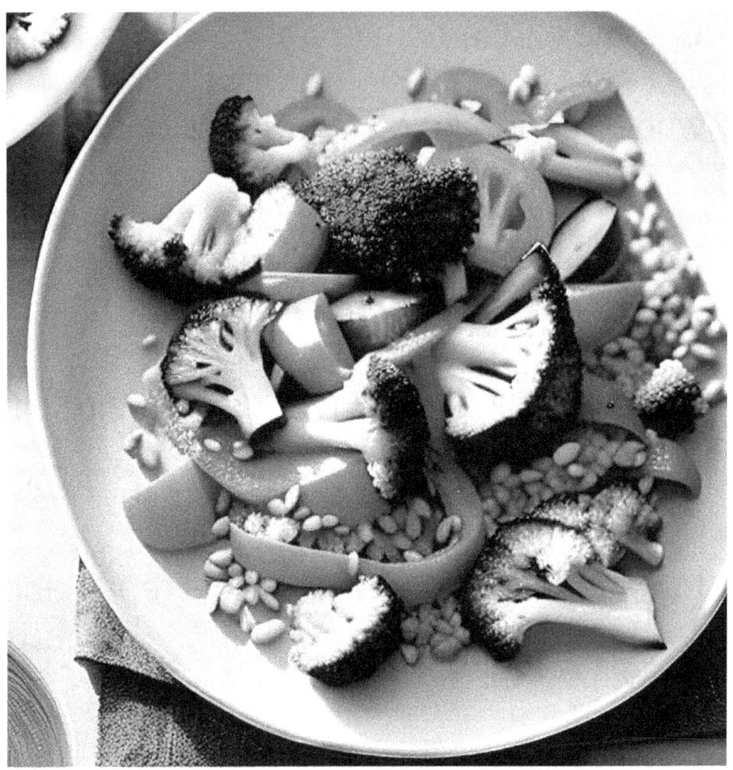

These provide critical vitamins, minerals, and antioxidants that aid in recuperation and overall health.

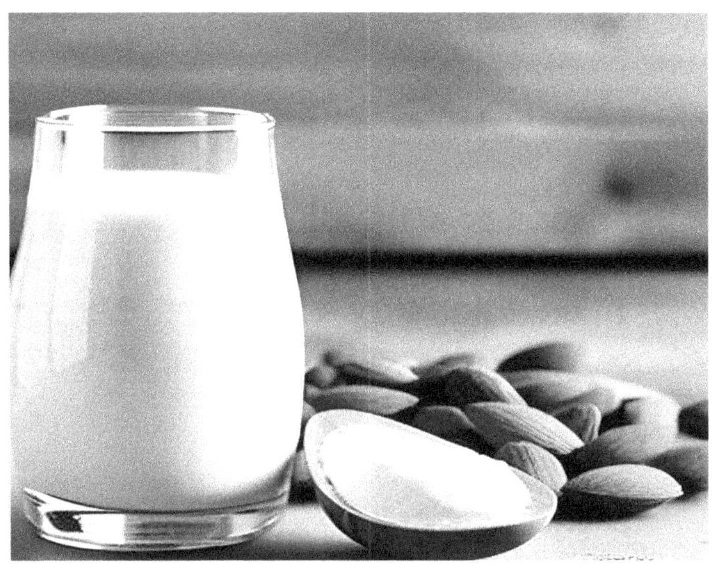

Dairy or Dairy Alternatives:

Low-fat dairy or fortified dairy alternatives (such as almond milk or soy milk) are good sources of calcium and vitamin D for bone health.

Post-Workout Snacks: After exercise, consider a snack containing both carbohydrates and protein, like a banana with peanut butter or yogurt with berries, to aid with recuperation.

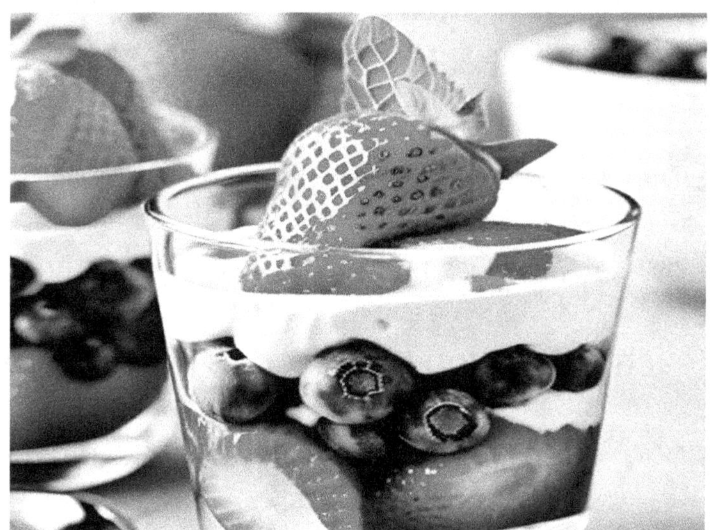

# Chapter 8

## Overcoming Common Challenges:

A. Dealing with Aches and Pains: As we age, it's natural to have aches and pains, especially when indulging in exercise. However, these discomforts shouldn't prevent you from being active. Here's how to manage and reduce aches and pains:

Proper Warm-Up: Ensure you complete a thorough warm-up before exercise to boost blood flow to your muscles and joints, lowering the probability of stiffness and soreness.

Listen to Your Body: Pay heed to your body's suggestions throughout your activity. If you suffer pain beyond typical muscle tiredness, quit the exercise immediately to prevent damage.

Stretching: Incorporate easy stretching exercises into your routine to reduce muscle tension and increase flexibility.

Rest and recovery: Give your body time to recover between sessions.

Overtraining can lead to increased aches and pains.

Hydration: Staying well hydrated will help prevent muscle cramps, which are prevalent among seniors.

B. Staying Motivated:

Maintaining motivation for exercise might be tough, but there are techniques to keep you inspired and devoted to your fitness routine:

Set realistic goals. Celebrate your victories along the way to keep motivated.

Variety: Change up your routines periodically to prevent boredom. Try new workouts, join fitness classes, or explore alternative physical hobbies.

Social Support: The social aspect can make training more pleasurable and create accountability.

Tracking Progress: Keep a fitness log to monitor your progress. Seeing increases in your strength, flexibility, or endurance can be immensely motivating.

Visualize Success: Imagine the benefits of regular exercise, such as improved health, higher vitality, and enhanced well-being, to stay motivated.

Reward Yourself: Treat yourself to tiny rewards as you hit key milestones. These rewards can operate as positive reinforcement.

C. Seeking Medical Advice When Necessary:

Your health and safety should always come first. If you encounter any of the following scenarios, it's crucial to get medical advice:

Chronic discomfort: If you feel chronic or severe discomfort during or after exercise, visit a healthcare expert. This could signal an underlying issue that needs to be addressed.

abrupt health changes: If you detect abrupt changes in your health, such as dizziness, shortness of breath, chest pain, or irregular heartbeats while exercising, stop immediately and seek medical help.

Chronic health illnesses: If you have pre-existing medical illnesses such as heart disease, diabetes, or arthritis, check with your healthcare professional before starting a new exercise regimen. They can provide recommendations on safe and acceptable activities.

Medication Adjustments: If you're taking medication, check with your healthcare practitioner to ensure that your workout program doesn't interfere with your prescription or require any adjustments.

Exercise-Related Injuries: If you incur an injury during exercise, no matter how small it may seem, visit a healthcare expert for proper examination and treatment.

Age-Related Changes: As your body undergoes age-related changes, consider regular check-ups with your healthcare practitioner to discuss any adjustments needed in your exercise plan.

Prioritizing your health and well-being is paramount. While exercise has several benefits, safety always comes first. Don't hesitate to seek medical counsel when necessary to ensure that you can continue your fitness journey safely and successfully.

# Chapter 9

## Social and Emotional Well-Being

A. Benefits of Exercise on Mental Health:

Exercise isn't just excellent for your physical health; it also has a profound impact on your mental well-being, which is especially vital for seniors over 60. Here are some ways exercise might benefit your mental health:

Mood Enhancement: Exercise causes the production of endorphins, frequently referred to as "feel-good" hormones, which can raise your mood and reduce symptoms of despair and anxiety.

Stress Reduction: Physical activity can help you manage and lower stress levels, generating a sense of relaxation and overall emotional well-being.

Improved Sleep: Regular exercise can contribute to higher sleep quality, helping you feel more refreshed and cognitively awake during the day.

Enhanced Cognitive Function: Exercise has been found to support cognitive function and memory, potentially lowering the risk of age-related cognitive decline.

Increased Confidence: Achieving fitness objectives, no matter how minor, can boost self-esteem and confidence.

Social Interaction: Engaging in group workouts or physical activities can provide opportunities for social interaction, lowering feelings of isolation and loneliness.

B. Group fitness options for seniors: Participating in group fitness activities can offer a sense of camaraderie and inspiration. Here are some group fitness choices ideal for seniors:

Senior Fitness Sessions: Many community centers, gyms, and senior centers offer personalized fitness sessions created exclusively for older people. These classes frequently involve low-impact aerobic, strength training, and flexibility exercises.

Yoga and Tai Chi: These mind-body disciplines not only promote physical flexibility and balance but also relaxation and stress reduction. Look for classes oriented toward elders.

Dance Classes: Dancing is a wonderful way to stay active and social. Consider classes in ballroom dancing, line dancing, or even Zumba, which can be customized for various fitness levels.

Walking Groups: Joining a local walking group is a fantastic way to enjoy the outdoors, get active, and interact with others in your neighborhood.

Water Aerobics: Water aerobics lessons are mild on the joints and provide a supportive and buoyant atmosphere for exercising.

Senior Sports Leagues: Some towns provide senior sports leagues for activities like golf, tennis, or pickleball, which provide both physical and social benefits.

C. Building a Supportive Network:

A supportive network of friends and family can significantly contribute to your general well-being. Here's how to create and strengthen your support network:

Stay Connected: Maintain regular touch with loved ones through phone calls, visits, or social media to strengthen relationships.

Join clubs or organizations: Participate in clubs, organizations, or groups that fit with your interests and hobbies, whether it's gardening, reading, or volunteer work.

Engage in community activities: Attend community events, classes, or workshops to meet like-minded folks and increase your social network.

Share Your Interests: When you engage in physical activities or workout classes, you're likely to meet people who share similar interests, offering an opportunity for interaction.

Seek Support: Don't hesitate to call on friends and family for support when required, whether it's for emotional support, transportation to fitness courses, or workout buddies.

Stay open to new connections: Be open to developing new connections at any age. Building connections and a supportive network can benefit your life in numerous ways.

# Conclusion

A. Summarizing Key Takeaways:

In this complete guide to "Easy Home Exercises for Seniors Over 60," we've addressed the important factors of maintaining a healthy and active lifestyle as you age. Here are the major takeaways:

Importance of Exercise: Regular exercise is vital for sustaining physical and mental health as a senior. Safe Home Workouts: You can engage in effective, safe workouts at home with the correct instruction and equipment. Exercise range: Incorporating a range of activities, including strength, balance, flexibility, and aerobic training, is vital to holistic fitness.

Proper Nutrition: A balanced diet and proper hydration are vital to fueling your body for exercise and overall well-being.

Social and Emotional Well-Being: Exercise not only benefits your physical health but also plays a key role in enhancing mental health and creating social connections.

Overcoming Challenges: Addressing aches and pains, keeping motivated, and getting medical guidance when necessary are key components of your fitness journey.

B. Encouraging a Lifelong Commitment to Fitness:

Your road toward better health and well-being doesn't have to stop here; it should continue as a lifelong commitment.

Embrace these principles:

Consistency: Stay dedicated to regular exercise, even when you experience obstacles and changes in your life.

Flexibility: Adapt your workout regimens to fit your changing demands and abilities.Seek Professional Guidance: Consider engaging fitness gurus, healthcare doctors, or physical therapists for specialized recommendations.

Enjoyment: Find activities you actually enjoy, as this will make it simpler to stay active throughout your life.Social Connection: Continue nurturing social connections, as they play a critical role in your general well-being.

Additional Resources and References:

To help your fitness journey, try exploring more tools and references:

Fitness applications and websites: There are various applications and websites that offer fitness routines, tracking tools, and instructional videos specialized for seniors. Community Programs: Check with local community centers, senior centers, or gyms for fitness programs geared for older people. Healthcare Providers: Consult your healthcare provider for personalized guidance on exercise and general health. Nutrition Resources: Explore resources on balanced diets and nutrition to complement your fitness endeavors. Support Groups: Consider joining support groups or online communities of seniors who share your fitness objectives and experiences. Remember that your health and well-being are lifelong endeavors, and by embracing exercise, nutrition, and social contacts, you can have a vibrant and rewarding senior life. Thank you for choosing to prioritize your health and fitness, and here's to many healthy and active years ahead!

# Appendices

A. Exercise Tracking Templates:

Staying organized and tracking your exercise progress is an excellent way to monitor your fitness journey. In this section, you'll find exercise tracking templates designed specifically for seniors over 60. These templates allow you to record your workouts, track improvements, and stay motivated as you achieve your fitness goals. Use them to log your strength training sessions, cardio workouts, flexibility routines, and more.


B. Recipes for Senior-Friendly Meals:

Maintaining a balanced diet is vital for your health and well-being. This section provides a collection of senior-friendly recipes that prioritize nutrition, taste, and ease of preparation. Whether you're looking for quick and nutritious breakfast options, flavorful lunch ideas, or satisfying dinners, these recipes offer a variety of choices to suit your dietary needs. Additionally, you'll find tips on meal planning and ingredient substitutions to accommodate specific dietary restrictions or preferences.

C. Glossary of Terms:

Fitness and exercise terminology can sometimes be confusing. In this glossary, you'll find definitions and explanations of common fitness and exercise terms. Whether you're new to exercise or looking to expand your understanding of fitness concepts, this resource will help you navigate the terminology used in the world of fitness and wellness. From words related to exercise types and techniques to nutritional terms, this glossary serves as a handy reference guide for all your fitness-related questions.

These appendices are designed to complement the information provided in the main chapters of this book. They serve as practical tools to assist you on your fitness journey, whether you're tracking your progress, preparing nutritious meals, or clarifying exercise-related terminology. Feel free to utilize these resources as you embark on your path to improved health and fitness.